About the NCCN Guidelines for Patients®

NCCN National Comprehensive Cancer Network®

AF824558

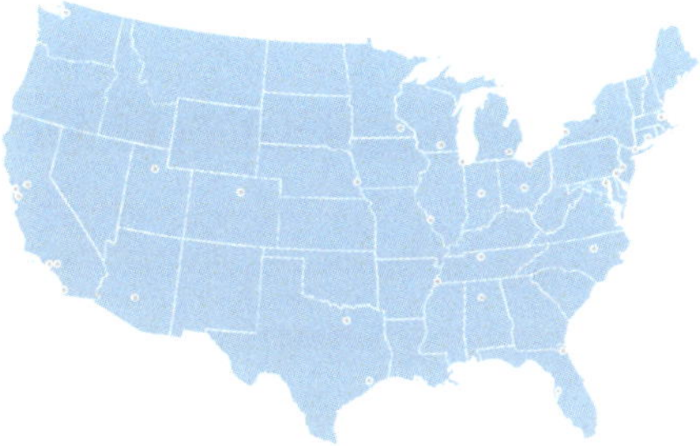

Did you know that top cancer centers across the United States work together to improve cancer care? This alliance of leading cancer centers is called the National Comprehensive Cancer Network® (NCCN®).

Cancer care is always changing. NCCN develops evidence-based cancer care recommendations used by health care providers worldwide. These frequently updated recommendations are the NCCN Clinical Practice Guidelines in Oncology (NCCN Guidelines®). The NCCN Guidelines for Patients plainly explain these expert recommendations for people with cancer and caregivers.

These NCCN Guidelines for Patients are based on the NCCN Clinical Practice Guidelines in Oncology (NCCN Guidelines®) for Breast Cancer Version 1.2024 – January 25, 2024.

View the NCCN Guidelines for Patients free online
NCCN.org/patientguidelines

Find an NCCN Cancer Center near you
NCCN.org/cancercenters

Connect with us YouTube

Supporters

NATIONAL COMPREHENSIVE CANCER NETWORK®
NCCN FOUNDATION
Guiding Treatment. Changing Lives.

NCCN Guidelines for Patients are supported by funding from the NCCN Foundation®

NCCN Foundation gratefully acknowledges the following corporate supporters for helping to make available these NCCN Guidelines for Patients: AstraZeneca and The Wawa Foundation.

NCCN independently adapts, updates, and hosts the NCCN Guidelines for Patients. Our corporate supporters do not participate in the development of the NCCN Guidelines for Patients and are not responsible for the content and recommendations contained therein.

To make a gift or learn more, visit online or email

NCCNFoundation.org/donate

PatientGuidelines@NCCN.org

Contents

4 Breast cancer basics

8 Testing for DCIS

19 Treating DCIS

32 Your treatment options

39 The breast after surgery

44 Making treatment decisions

55 Words to know

59 NCCN Contributors

60 NCCN Cancer Centers

62 Index

NCCN Foundation seeks to support the millions of patients and their families affected by a cancer diagnosis by funding and distributing NCCN Guidelines for Patients. NCCN Foundation is also committed to advancing cancer treatment by funding the nation's promising doctors at the center of innovation in cancer research. For more details and the full library of patient and caregiver resources, visit NCCN.org/patients.

National Comprehensive Cancer Network (NCCN) and NCCN Foundation
3025 Chemical Road, Suite 100, Plymouth Meeting, PA 19462 USA

1

Breast cancer basics

5 The breast

6 Ductal carcinoma in situ

7 Key points

Ductal carcinoma in situ (DCIS) is found in the cells that line the ducts in the breast. DCIS is stage 0 or noninvasive cancer. This means the cancerous cells are in place (in situ) and have not spread outside the ducts. DCIS is treated to prevent invasive breast cancer, a more advanced form of cancer.

The breast

The breast is an organ and a gland found on the chest. The breast is made of milk ducts, fat, nerves, lymph and blood vessels, ligaments, and other connective tissue. Behind the breast is the pectoral (chest) muscle and ribs. Muscle and ligaments help hold the breast in place.

Breast tissue contains glands that can make milk. These milk glands are called lobules. Lobules look like tiny clusters of grapes. Small tubes called ducts connect the lobules to the nipple.

The ring of darker breast skin is called the areola. The raised tip within the areola is called the nipple. The nipple-areola complex (NAC) is a term that refers to both parts.

The breast

The breast is a glandular organ made up of milk ducts, fat, nerves, blood and lymph vessels, ligaments, and other connective tissue.

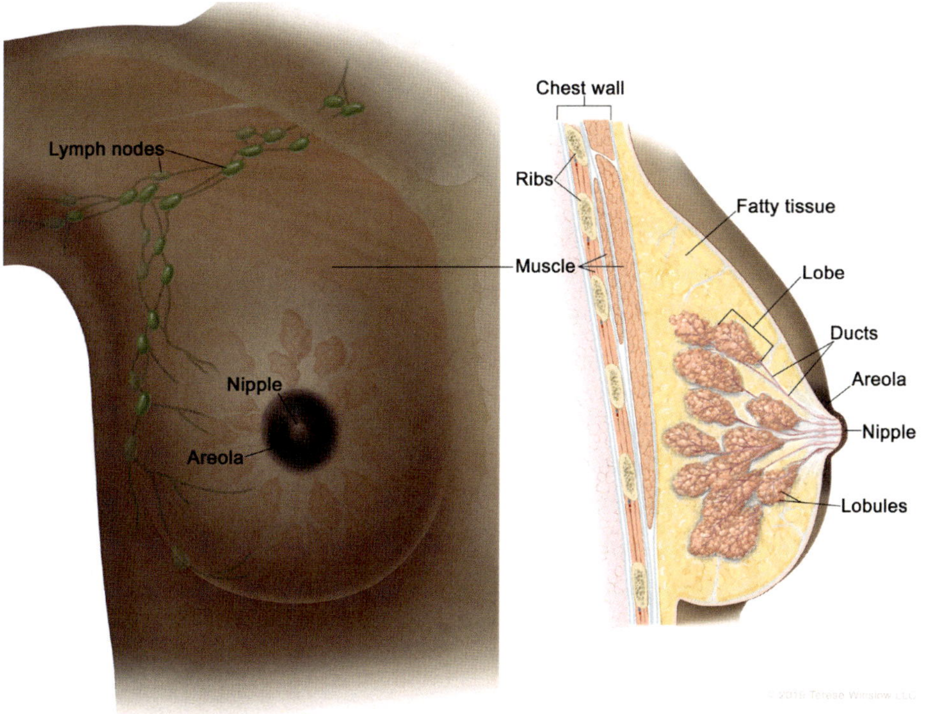

Lymph fluid drains from breast tissue into lymph vessels and travels to lymph nodes near your armpit (axilla). Lymphatic fluid is a clear fluid that gives cells water and food. It also helps to fight germs. Nodes near the armpit are called axillary lymph nodes (ALNs).

Ductal carcinoma in situ

Ductal carcinoma in situ (DCIS) or intraductal carcinoma is found in the cells that line the ducts. Ducts are thin tubes that carry milk in the breast. DCIS is noninvasive cancer. Noninvasive means the cancerous cells are in place (in situ) and have not spread anywhere else.

DCIS is a preinvasive disease. DCIS is treated to prevent invasive breast cancer, a more advanced form of cancer. Invasive breast cancer is breast cancer that has spread from the milk ducts or milk glands (lobules) into the surrounding breast tissue or nearby lymph nodes. Once outside the ducts or lobules, breast cancer can spread through lymph or blood to lymph nodes or other parts of the body.

Anyone can develop breast cancer, including those assigned male at birth. Although there are some differences between those assigned male and those assigned female at birth, treatment is very similar for all genders.

DCIS

Ductal carcinoma in situ (DCIS) is found in the cells that line the thin tubes (ducts) that carry milk to the breast. The cancerous cells are in place (in situ) and have not spread.

Ductal Carcinoma In Situ (DCIS)

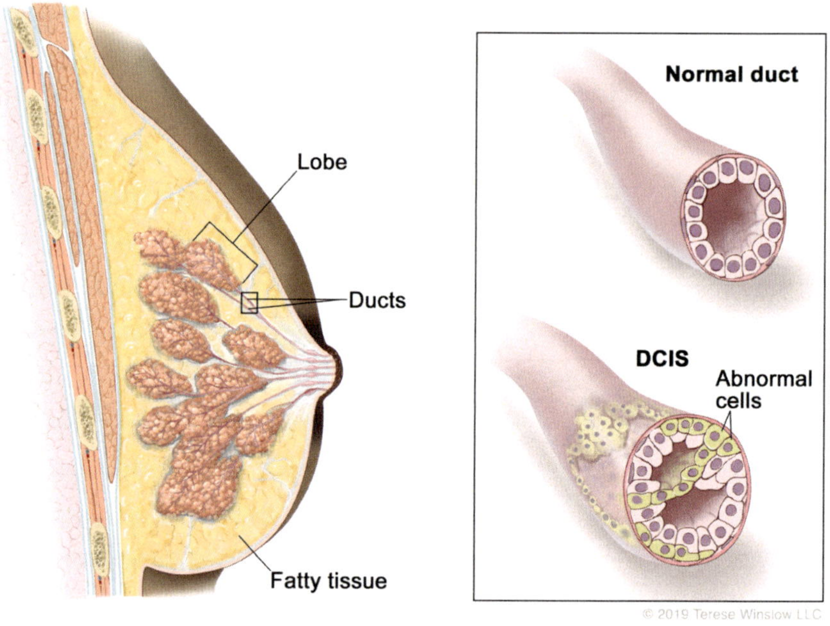

Key points

- Anyone can develop breast cancer.
- Inside breasts are lobules, ducts, fat, blood and lymph vessels, ligaments, and connective tissue. Lobules are structures that make breast milk. Ducts carry breast milk from the lobules to the nipple.
- Breast cancer often starts in the ducts or lobules and then spreads into the surrounding tissue.
- Cancerous cells found only inside the ducts or lobules is called noninvasive. Ductal carcinoma in situ (DCIS) is found only in the ducts.
- Invasive breast cancer is cancer that has grown outside the ducts or lobules into surrounding tissue. Once outside the ducts or lobules, breast cancer can spread through lymph or blood to lymph nodes or other parts of the body.

What's the difference between a screening and diagnostic mammogram?

A mammogram is a picture of the inside of your breast made using x-rays. During a mammogram, the breast is pressed between two plates while you stand in different positions. Multiple x-rays will be taken. A computer combines the x-rays to make detailed pictures.

- Screening mammograms are done on a regular basis when there are no signs or symptoms of breast cancer. Results take a few days.
- Diagnostic mammograms are used for those who have symptoms such as a lump, pain, nipple thickening or discharge, or whose breasts have changed shape or size.
- Diagnostic mammograms are also used to take a closer look at an abnormal area found in a screening mammogram.
- A radiologist will evaluate the diagnostic mammogram while you wait so if additional testing is needed, it can be done right away.
- Both types of mammograms use low-dose x-rays to examine the breast. They may use either the standard 2-dimensional (2D) digital mammogram or 3-dimensional (3D) mammogram known as tomosynthesis.

2

Testing for DCIS

9 Test results

10 General health tests

10 Physical exam

11 Imaging tests

12 Biopsy

14 Estrogen receptor status

15 Genetic cancer risk testing

16 Cancer stages

18 Key points

Treatment planning starts with testing. This chapter presents an overview of the tests you might receive and what to expect.

Test results

Results from biopsy and imaging studies will be used to determine your treatment plan. Treatment will be based on these findings. It is important you understand what these tests mean. Ask questions and keep copies of your test results.

Keep these things in mind:

- Choose a friend, family member, or peer who can drive you to appointments, provide meals, or offer emotional support during diagnosis and treatment.
- Bring someone with you to doctor visits, if possible.
- Write down questions and take notes during appointments. Don't be afraid to ask your care team questions. Get to know your care team and help them get to know you.
- Get copies of blood tests, imaging results, and reports about the specific type of cancer you have.
- Organize your papers. Create files for insurance forms, medical records, and test results. You can do the same on your computer.
- Keep a list of contact information for everyone on your care team. Add it to your phone. Hang the list on your refrigerator or keep it in a place where someone can access it in an emergency. Keep your primary care physician (PCP) informed of changes to this list. You are encouraged to keep your PCP in the loop. They are great partners in your care.
- In your contact list, include information on the exact type of cancer you have, as well as any treatments you've received and the date each treatment started.
- Set up a MyChart or health record account if it's available, which can help you track your appointments and communicate with your care team.

For possible tests, **see Guide 1.**

Guide 1 Possible tests
Medical history and physical exam
Diagnostic mammogram
Biopsy with pathology review
Determine estrogen receptor (ER) status
Genetic counseling, if at risk for hereditary breast cancer
Breast MRI or ultrasound, as needed

General health tests

Medical history

A medical history is a record of all health issues and treatments you have had in your life. Be prepared to list any illness or injury and when it happened. Bring a list of old and new medicines and any over-the-counter (OTC) medicines, herbals, or supplements you take. Some supplements interact and affect medicines that your care team may prescribe. Tell your care team about any symptoms you have. A medical history, sometimes called a health history, will help determine which treatment is best for you.

Family history

Some cancers and other diseases can run in families. Your care team will ask about the health history of family members who are blood relatives. This information is called a family history. Ask family members on both sides of your family about their health issues like heart disease, cancer, and diabetes, and at what age they were diagnosed. It's important to know the specific type of cancer or where the cancer started, if it is in multiple locations, and if they had genetic testing.

Physical exam

During a physical exam, your health care provider may:

- Check your temperature, blood pressure, pulse, and breathing rate
- Check your height and weight
- Listen to your lungs and heart
- Look in your eyes, ears, nose, and throat
- Feel and apply pressure to parts of your body to see if organs are of normal size, are soft or hard, or cause pain when touched.
- Examine your breasts to look for lumps, nipple discharge or bleeding, or skin changes.
- Feel for enlarged lymph nodes in your neck, underarm, and groin.

Clinical breast exam

Clinical breast exam (CBE) is a physical exam of the bare breast performed by a health care provider to check for lumps or other changes. It is done while you are seated and/or lying down. Your provider should take time to palpate (feel) the entire breast, including the armpit. A nurse or assistant might also be in the room during the exam.

Imaging tests

Imaging tests take pictures of the inside of your body. Imaging tests show the primary tumor, or where the cancer started, and look for cancer in other parts of the body.

A radiologist, an expert in interpreting imaging tests, will write a report and send this report to your doctor. It is likely that the report will be sent directly to you through your patient portal or patient access system. Your care team should discuss these results you.

Diagnostic mammogram

A mammogram is a picture of the inside of your breast. The picture is made using x-rays. A computer combines the x-rays to make detailed pictures. Mammogram results are used to plan treatment.

Diagnostic mammograms look at specific areas of your breasts, which may not be clearly seen on screening mammograms. They are used to see tumor and the size of the tumor(s). Diagnostic mammograms include extra compression in certain areas of the breast, magnification views, or rolling the breast to image additional areas of the breast. Other diagnostic tests may include a breast MRI or ultrasound (US).

Contrast material

Contrast materials are not dyes, but substances that help make the pictures of the inside of the body clearer. The contrast is not permanent and will leave the body in your urine after the test. There is more than one type of contrast and it differs depending on the test. Tell your care team if you have had allergic reactions to contrast in the past. This is important. You might be given medicines to avoid the effects of those allergies.

Contrast-enhanced mammogram

Contrast-enhanced mammography is a new technology that uses contrast material to improve the pictures of the inside of the breast. It is sometimes used for those who cannot have a MRI scan.

Breast MRI

A magnetic resonance imaging (MRI) scan uses radio waves and powerful magnets to take pictures of the inside of the body. It does not use radiation. If needed, an MRI would be used in addition to a mammogram. Because of the very strong magnets used in the MRI machine, tell the technologist if you have any metal in your body.

For a breast MRI, a gadolinium-based contrast agent (GBCA)—a rare, heavy metal—is used to enhance the quality of the MRI. There are no harmful effects from GBCA, but it may linger in the body for months to years afterward. Talk to your doctor if you have any concerns.

Ultrasound

An ultrasound (US) uses high-energy sound waves to form pictures of the inside of the body. This is similar to the sonogram used for pregnancy. A wand-like probe (transducer) will be held and moved on your bare breast using gel. It may also be placed below your armpit. Ultrasound does not use x-rays. It is good at showing small areas of cancer that are near the skin. Sometimes, a breast ultrasound or MRI is used to guide a biopsy.

Biopsy

A biopsy is a procedure that removes a sample of tissue or fluid. The sample is sent to a lab for testing. A pathologist will examine the biopsy for cancer and write a report called a pathology report. Ask questions about your biopsy results and what they mean for your treatment.

There are different types of biopsies. Some biopsies are guided using imaging, such as mammogram, ultrasound, or MRI. The primary or main tumor is biopsied first. Other tumors or tumors in different areas may also be biopsied. You may have tissue removed from the breast, lymph nodes, or both.

Types of possible biopsies include:

- **Fine-needle aspiration (FNA) or core biopsy (CB)** uses needles of different sizes to remove a sample of tissue or fluid. In a vacuum-assisted core biopsy (VACB), suction is used through a needle to remove the sample using a special vacuum device.
- **Incisional biopsy** removes a small amount of tissue through a small cut in the skin or body.
- **Excisional biopsy** removes the entire abnormal area. This is not the preferred type of biopsy but may be necessary if other methods are not possible or when the biopsy results don't match the expected findings. This is usually done under anesthesia in an operating room.

Standard of care is the best-known way to treat a particular disease based on past clinical trials. There may be more than one treatment regimen that is considered standard of care. Ask your care team what treatment options are available and if a clinical trial might be right for you.

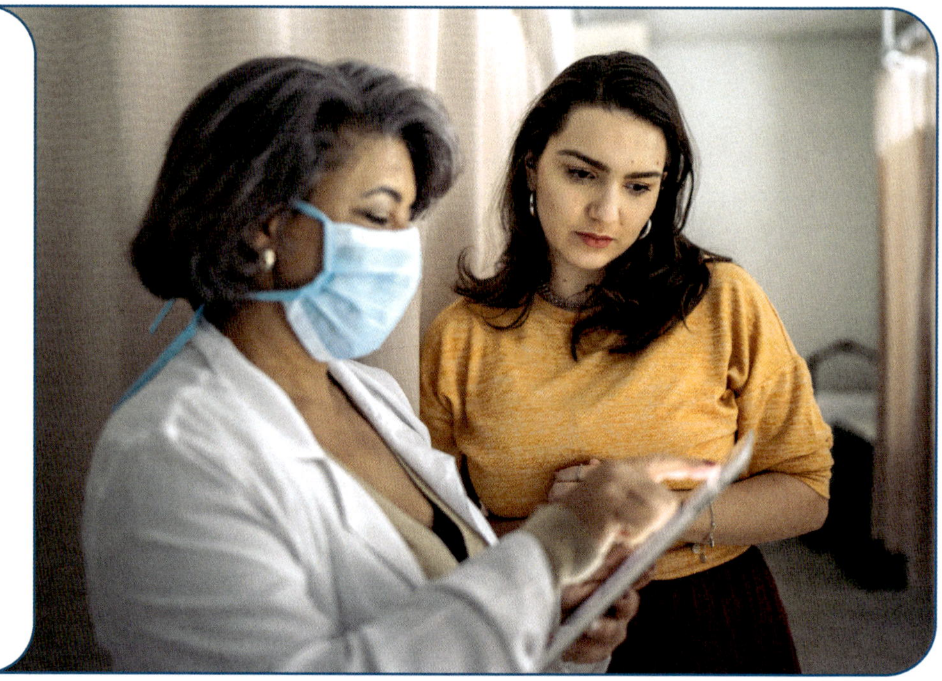

Before biopsies are performed, usually the area is injected with numbing medicine. A core needle biopsy (CNB) removes more than one tissue sample, but usually through the same area on the breast. The samples are small. The needle is often guided into the tumor with imaging. When mammography is used during a biopsy, it is called a stereotactic needle biopsy.

One or more clips may be placed near the breast tumor during a biopsy. The clips are small, painless, and made of metal. They will mark the site for future treatment and imaging. The clips stay in place until surgery. If the area biopsied is benign, the clip will remain in place to mark the biopsy site on future imaging. The clips cause no problems, even if they are left in place for a long time. You will be able to go through airport security and have an MRI with the clip(s) in place.

There are both physical and emotional experiences in having biopsies. You may need to rest and place an ice pack on the biopsy area after the procedure. If you are working or have other commitments, you may want to take the day off to rest.

Biopsy results

Histology is the study of the anatomy (structure) of cells, tissues, and organs under a microscope. It is used to make treatment decisions. Your pathology report will contain information about histology.

You may be recommended to have an open biopsy (surgery) to remove (excise) the tumor to confirm histology. Talk to your health care provider for more information on next steps.

Biopsy

In a biopsy, a sample of tumor is removed. There are different types of biopsy. This image shows an ultrasound-guided needle biopsy.

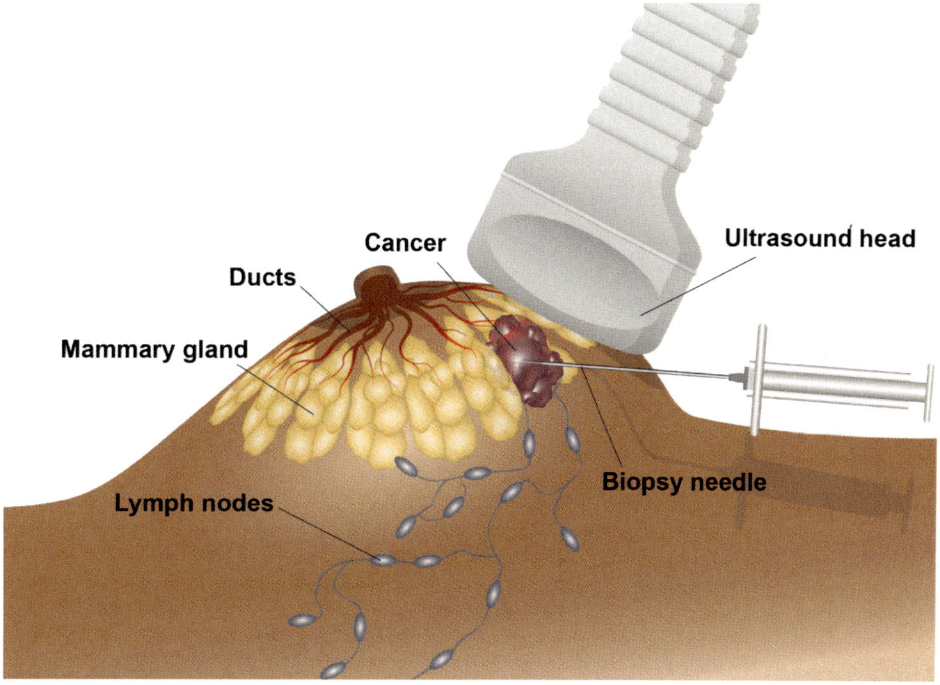

Estrogen receptor status

Estrogen is a hormone that plays a role in breast development. A hormone is a substance made by a gland in your body. Your blood carries hormones throughout your body. A receptor is a protein found inside or on the surface of a cell. Substances such as hormones attach (bind) to these receptors. This causes changes within the cell.

Hormones recognize and bind to specific hormone receptors. When hormones, such as estrogen, attach to receptors inside breast cancer cells, they can cause cancer to grow. If found, these estrogen receptors may be targeted for treatment using endocrine therapy.

Immunohistochemistry

Immunohistochemistry (IHC) is a special staining process that involves adding a chemical marker to cells. These cells are then studied using a microscope. IHC can find estrogen receptors in breast cancer cells. A pathologist will measure how many cells have estrogen receptors and the number of estrogen receptors inside each cell. Test results will either be estrogen receptor-positive (ER+) or estrogen receptor-negative (ER-).

HER2 testing is not used in the diagnosis and treatment of DCIS.

Estrogen receptor-positive

In estrogen receptor-positive (ER+) breast cancer, IHC finds estrogen hormone receptors in at least 1 out of every 100 cancer cells. ER+ cancer cells may need estrogen to grow. These cells may stop growing or die with endocrine treatment to block estrogen production or estrogen receptor signaling.

Estrogen receptor-negative

Estrogen receptor-negative (ER-) breast cancer cells do not have estrogen hormone receptors. These cancer cells do not need estrogen to grow and continue to grow. Therefore, estrogen-blocking treatment is not effective.

Genetic cancer risk testing

About 1 out of 10 breast cancers are hereditary. Depending on your family history or other features of your cancer, your health care provider might refer you for hereditary genetic testing to learn more about your cancer. A genetic counselor or trained provider will speak to you about the results. Tests results may be used to guide treatment planning.

Genetic testing is done collecting blood or saliva (spitting into a cup or a cheek swab). The goal is to look for gene mutations inherited from your biological parents called germline mutations. Some mutations can put you at risk for more than one type of cancer. You can pass these genes on to your children. Also, other blood relatives might carry these mutations. Tell your care team if there is a family history of cancer.

BRCA tests

Everyone has *BRCA* genes. Normal *BRCA* genes help to prevent tumor growth. They help fix damaged cells and help cells grow normally. *BRCA* mutations put you at risk for more than one type of cancer. Mutations in *BRCA1* or *BRCA2* increase the risk of breast, ovarian, prostate, colorectal, pancreatic, and melanoma skin cancers. Mutated *BRCA* genes can also affect how well some treatments work. These tests might be repeated to help determine the best treatment.

What is your family health history?

Some cancers and other diseases run in families—those who are related to you through genes passed down from biological parent to child. This information is called a family health history. Ask blood relatives about their health issues like heart disease, cancer, and diabetes, and at what age they were diagnosed. For relatives who were diagnosed with cancer, ask them (or other relatives if they are no longer living) what type of cancer they had, if they died from the cancer, and at what age the cancer was diagnosed.

Start by asking your parents, siblings, and children. Next, talk to half-siblings, aunts and uncles, nieces and nephews, grandparents, and grandchildren.

Write down what you learn about your family history and share with your health care provider.

Some of the questions to ask include:

- ✓ How old were you when each of these diseases and health conditions was diagnosed?
- ✓ What is our family's ancestry—from what countries did our ancestors originate?

Cancer stages

Breast cancer staging is often done twice.

- **Clinical stage (c)** is the rating given before any treatment. It is based on a physical exam, biopsy, and imaging tests. An example might look like cT0 or cN1.
- **Pathologic stage (p)** or surgical stage is determined by examining tissue removed during surgery. An example might be pT1.

A cancer stage is a way to describe the extent of the cancer at the time you are first diagnosed. The American Joint Committee on Cancer (AJCC) created a staging system to determine how much cancer is in your body, where it is located, and what subtype you have. AJCC is just one type of staging system.

Staging is based on a combination of information to reach a final numbered stage. Often, not all information is available at the initial evaluation. More information can be gathered as treatment begins.

TNM scores

The tumor, node, metastasis (TNM) system is used to stage breast cancer. In this system, the letters T, N, and M describe different areas of cancer growth. Based on imaging and pathology results, a score or number is assigned to each letter. The higher the number, the larger the tumor or the more the cancer has spread. These scores will be combined to assign the cancer a stage. A TNM example might look like this: T1N0M0 or T1, N0, M0, or for DCIS TisN0M0.

- **T (tumor)** – Depth and spread of the main (primary) tumor(s) in one or both breasts
- **N (node)** – If cancer has spread to nearby (regional) lymph nodes
- **M (metastasis)** – If cancer has spread to distant parts of the body or metastasized

Lymph nodes

Lymphatic fluid, a clear fluid containing cells that help fight infections and other diseases, drains through channels into lymphatic vessels. From here, lymph drains into lymph nodes. Lymph nodes work as filters to help fight infection. Regional lymph nodes are found near the breast in the armpit (axilla). If breast cancer spreads, it often goes first to nearby lymph nodes under the arm. It can also sometimes spread to lymph nodes near the collarbone or near the breastbone. However, it is possible for cancerous cells to travel through lymph and blood to other parts of the body without having gone to the lymph nodes first.

Grade

Grade describes how abnormal the tumor cells look under a microscope (called histology). Higher-grade cancers tend to grow and spread faster than lower-grade cancers. GX means the grade can't be determined, followed by G1, G2, and G3. G3 is the highest grade for breast cancers.

- **GX** – Grade cannot be determined
- **G1** – Low (nuclear grade 1)
- **G2** – Intermediate (nuclear grade 2)
- **G3** – High (nuclear grade 3)

Numbered stages

Numbered stages are based on TNM scores. Stages range from stage 0 to stage 4, with 4 being the most advanced. They might be written as stage 0, stage I, stage II, stage III, and stage IV. For example, DCIS is stage 0 or Tis, N0, M0.

- **Stage 0 is noninvasive** – Noninvasive breast cancer is rated stage 0. DCIS is found only in the ducts (Tis). It has not spread to the surrounding breast tissue, lymph nodes (N0), or distant sites (M0).
- **Stages 1, 2, and 3 are invasive** – Invasive breast cancer is rated stage 1, 2, or 3. It has grown outside the ducts, lobules, or breast skin. Cancer might be in the axillary lymph nodes.
- **Stage 4 is metastatic** – Stage 4 breast cancer has spread to distant sites. It can develop from earlier stages or rarely, your first diagnosis can be stage 4 metastatic breast cancer (called de novo).

More information on invasive and metastatic breast cancers can be found at NCCN.org/patientguidelines and on the NCCN Patient Guides for Cancer app.

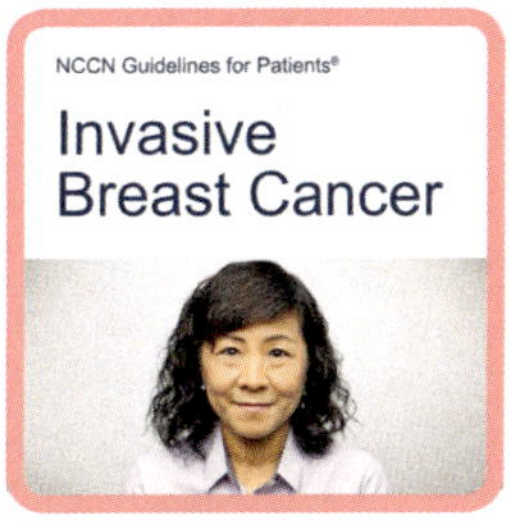

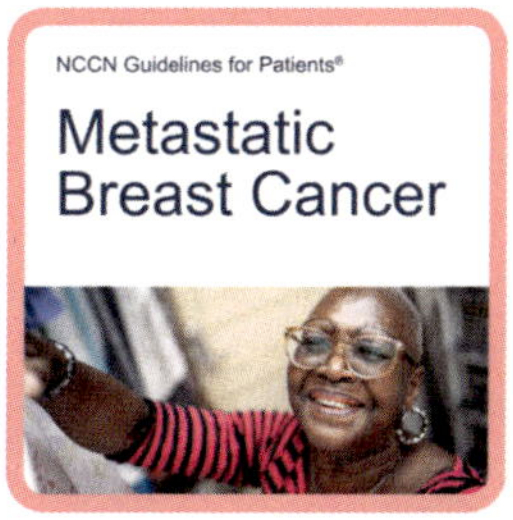

Key points

- Tests are used to find cancer, plan treatment, and check how well treatment is working.
- You will have a physical exam, including a breast exam, to see if anything feels or looks abnormal.
- A diagnostic mammogram includes detailed pictures of both breasts. It is different than a screening mammogram.
- During a biopsy, tissue or fluid samples are removed for testing. Samples are needed to confirm the presence of cancer and to perform cancer cell tests.
- Some breast cancers grow because of estrogen. Testing will be done to see if you have estrogen receptor-positive (ER+) breast cancer. This provides information about the behavior of your cancer, as well as treatments to which your cancer may respond.
- A cancer stage is a way to describe the extent of the cancer at the time you are first diagnosed. Breast cancer is often staged twice, before and after surgery.

Testing takes time. It might take days or weeks for all test results to come in.

3

Treating DCIS

20 Care team

22 Surgery

24 Radiation therapy

25 Endocrine therapy

27 Clinical trials

29 Supportive care

31 Key points

There is more than one treatment for DCIS. This chapter describes treatment options and what to expect. Together, you and your care team will choose a treatment plan that is best for you.

Care team

Treating breast cancer takes a team approach. Treatment decisions should involve a multidisciplinary team (MDT). An MDT is a team of health care and psychosocial care professionals from different professional backgrounds who have knowledge (expertise) and experience in your type of cancer. This team is united in the planning and implementing of your treatment. Ask who will coordinate your care.

Some members of your care team will be with you throughout cancer treatment, while others will only be there for parts of it. Get to know your care team and help them get to know you.

Depending on your diagnosis, the care team might include the following specialists:

- **Oncologists** are doctors who specialize in diagnosing and treating cancer. Types of oncologists include medical, radiation, and surgical oncologists.
- **A reconstructive (plastic) surgeon** performs oncoplastic (breast cancer surgery) reductions, balancing procedures, and breast reconstruction.
- **Oncology nurses** provide your hands-on care, like giving systemic therapy, managing your care, answering questions, and helping you cope with side effects.
- **Oncology pharmacists** are experts in knowing how to use medicines to treat cancer and to manage symptoms and side effects.
- **Nutritionists and dietitians** can provide guidance on what foods are most suitable for your condition.
- **An occupational therapist** helps people with the tasks of daily living.
- **A physical therapist** helps people move with greater comfort and ease.
- **A certified lymphedema therapist** gives a type of massage called manual lymph drainage.
- **Psychologists and psychiatrists** are mental health experts who can help manage issues such as depression, anxiety, or other mental health conditions that can affect how you think and feel.

- **Social workers** help people solve and cope with problems in their everyday lives. Clinical social workers also diagnose and treat mental, behavioral, and emotional issues. The anxiety a person feels when diagnosed with cancer might be managed by a social worker in some cancer centers. They, or other designated professionals, can help navigate the complexities of financial and insurance stresses.
- **Spiritual care specialists** identify and support those with spiritual distress or unmet spiritual needs.
- **Smoking cessation specialists** can provide medication and counseling for those who would like to stop using tobacco or nicotine products.
- **A research team** helps to collect research data and coordinate care if you are in a clinical trial. Clinical trials help bring new therapies to patients and advance the treatment for everyone. Consider asking your care team about access to clinical trials.

If you smoke or vape, seek help to quit

A history of smoking or vaping nicotine increases your chances of developing lung and other cancers. Smoking and vaping can limit how well cancer treatment works and prevent wound healing. They also greatly increase your chances of having side effects during and after surgery. Cannabis use might also affect the amount of anesthesia used during surgery.

Nicotine is the chemical in tobacco that makes you want to keep smoking and vaping. Nicotine withdrawal is challenging for most people who smoke or vape. The stress of having cancer may make it even harder to quit. If you smoke or vape, ask your care team about counseling and medicines to help you quit.

For online support, try these websites:

- SmokeFree.gov
- BeTobaccoFree.gov
- CDC.gov/tobacco

Surgery

Surgery is an operation or procedure to remove cancer from the body. Surgery is the main or primary treatment for DCIS. This is only one part of a treatment plan. When preparing for surgery, seek the opinion of an experienced surgeon. The surgeon should be an expert in performing your type of surgery. Hospitals that perform many surgeries often have better results. You can ask for a referral to a hospital or cancer center that has experience in treating your type of cancer.

Your preferences about treatment are always important. Make your wishes known.

Goal of surgery

The goal of surgery or tumor resection is to remove all the cancer. To do so, the tumor is removed along with a rim of normal-looking tissue around its edge called the surgical margin. The surgical margin may look normal during surgery, but cancerous cells may be found when viewed under a microscope by a pathologist. A clear or negative margin (R0) is when no cancer cells are found in the tissue around the edge of the tumor. In a positive margin, cancer cells are found in normal-looking tissue around the tumor.

After surgery, you may receive treatment such as radiation to kill any remaining cancer cells. You might have a wound drain to prevent fluid from collecting in the body after surgery. These drains are usually removed a few days after surgery.

Breast-conserving surgery

The dotted line shows where the tumor is removed. Lumpectomy is the removal of abnormal cells or tumor and not the whole breast. It is also called a partial mastectomy, breast-conserving therapy, or breast-conserving surgery (BCS).

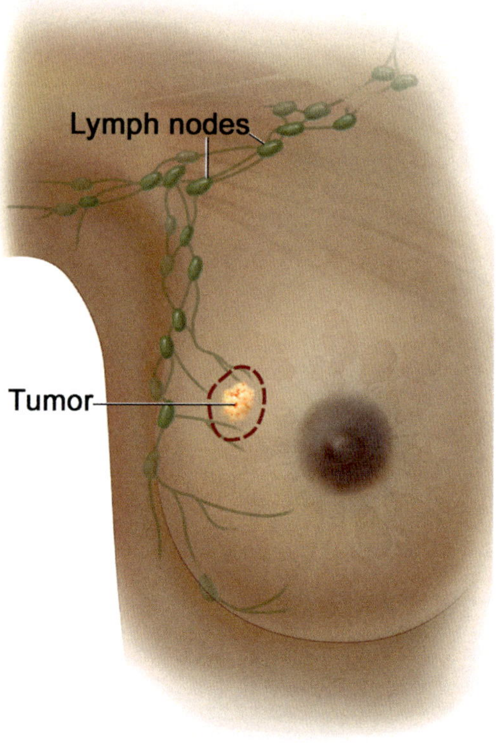

Lumpectomy

Lumpectomy is the removal of abnormal cells or tumor. It does not remove the whole breast. A lumpectomy is also called breast-conserving therapy or breast-conserving surgery (BCS). In a lumpectomy, the surgeon aims to remove all DCIS with a rim of healthy tissue around it, called a negative, or clear, surgical margin. Having a negative surgical margin will decrease the chance that cancer may return in that area of the breast. You may need more than one surgery to achieve negative margins and ensure all the cancer was removed. A lumpectomy is usually followed by radiation therapy to part of or the whole breast. It is important to note that a lymph node biopsy is not done with a lumpectomy.

The breast might not look the same after a lumpectomy. Speak to your surgeon about how a lumpectomy might affect the look and shape of your breast, and any concerns you have. You can also seek the opinion of a plastic surgeon.

Breastfeeding or chestfeeding

Breastfeeding or chestfeeding following a lumpectomy may be possible. However, after treatments, the breast may produce less milk than before, or none. Breastfeeding/chestfeeding is not recommended during active treatment or within 6 months of completing certain types of endocrine therapy.

Mastectomy

A mastectomy removes all of the breast. Before removing the breast, the surgeon may do a sentinel lymph node biopsy (SLNB). Sentinel lymph nodes (SLNs) are the first lymph nodes cancer cells are likely to have spread to from the primary tumor.

Types of mastectomies include:

- **A total mastectomy or simple mastectomy** removes the whole breast with a flat skin closure.
- **A skin-sparing mastectomy** removes the breast but not all of the skin, in order to have breast reconstruction that might include flaps and/or implants.
- **Nipple-sparing mastectomy** preserves the nipple-areola complex (NAC) as well as all of the skin. Not everyone is a candidate for nipple-sparing mastectomy based upon location of cancer, breast size, and breast ptosis (degree of drooping).

Breast reconstruction is an option after a mastectomy. It might be done at the same time as mastectomy (immediate) or at some time following the completion of cancer treatment (delayed). Breast reconstruction is most commonly done in stages. If you are considering breast reconstruction surgery, it requires collaboration between a breast surgeon and a reconstructive (plastic) surgeon.

Sentinel lymph node biopsy

A sentinel lymph node biopsy (SLNB or SNB) is done during a mastectomy to determine if any cancer cells have traveled to the lymph nodes. A sentinel lymph node (SLN) is the first lymph node or nodes that cancer cells are most likely to spread to from a primary tumor. Often, there is more than one sentinel lymph node. Just because these nodes are removed, it does not mean that they test positive for cancer.

To find the sentinel lymph nodes, a dye is injected into the breast. It may be a radioactive material, blue dye, or other tracer. The tracer travels through the lymph channels in the breast to the lymph nodes in the armpit. This helps the surgeon find which of the lymph nodes are the sentinel lymph nodes. The lymph nodes containing the tracer are removed and tested by a pathologist.

Radiation therapy

Radiation therapy (RT) uses high-energy radiation from x-rays (photons), protons, and other sources to kill any remaining cancer cells after surgery. Different types of radiation can be used for DCIS. Most types include several short treatment sessions that are given once daily over a few days to weeks. Ask your care team which radiation option(s) are best for you and what side effects to expect.

Types of radiation therapy used in DCIS include:

- **Whole breast radiation therapy (WBRT)** is used to treat the entire breast. Sometimes, additional treatments may be given to the tumor area. This is called a boost.
- **Partial breast irradiation (PBI)** is used to treat only the tumor area of the breast. Accelerated partial breast irradiation (APBI) is radiation given over a shorter period of time.

External beam radiation therapy

External beam radiation therapy (EBRT) uses a machine outside the body to aim radiation at the whole breast (WBRT) or only the tumor area of the breast (PBI).

Internal radiation

Internal radiation (brachytherapy) involves placing one or more small tubes into the tumor area of the breast. A small radioactive seed travels into the tube(s) and delivers radiation to the tumor area of the breast from inside the body. This type of radiation is used only for PBI.

Endocrine therapy

The endocrine system is made up of organs and tissues that produce hormones. Hormones are natural chemicals released into the bloodstream.

There are 4 hormones that might be targeted in endocrine therapy for breast cancer:

- **Estrogen** is made mainly by the ovaries, but is also made by other tissues in the body such as fat tissue.
- **Progesterone** is made mainly by the ovaries.
- **Luteinizing hormone-releasing hormone (LHRH)** is made by a part of the brain called the hypothalamus. It tells the ovaries to make estrogen and progesterone and testicles to make testosterone. LHRH is also called gonadotropin-releasing hormone (GnRH).
- **Androgen** is made by the adrenal glands, testicles, and ovaries.

Hormones may cause breast cancer to grow. Endocrine therapy will stop your body from making hormones or it will block what hormones do in the body. This can help to reduce the risk of cancer returning.

Endocrine therapy is sometimes called hormone therapy. It is not the same as hormone replacement therapy (HRT) used for menopause.

Types of endocrine therapy that might be used for DCIS:

- **Aromatase inhibitors (AIs)** stop a type of hormone called androgen from changing into estrogen by interfering with an enzyme called aromatase. They do not affect estrogen made by the ovaries. Non-steroidal aromatase inhibitors include anastrozole (Arimidex) and letrozole (Femara). Exemestane (Aromasin) is a steroidal aromatase inhibitor.
- **Estrogen receptor (ER) modulators** or anti-estrogens prevent hormones from binding to receptors.
- **Selective estrogen receptor modulators (SERMs)** block estrogen from attaching to hormone receptors. They include tamoxifen and toremifene (Fareston).
- **Selective estrogen receptor degraders (SERDs)** block and destroy estrogen receptors. Fulvestrant (Faslodex) and elacestrant (Orserdu) are SERDs.
- **Gonadotropin-releasing hormone (GnRH)** agonists might be used to suppress ovarian hormone or testosterone production.

Endocrine therapy will suppress the production of hormones and affect one's abilty to become pregnant during treatment. Those who want to have children in the future should be referred to a fertility specialist before starting endocrine therapy.

Testosterone

For those assigned male at birth whose bodies continue to make testosterone, endocrine therapy includes tamoxifen or an aromatase inhibitor with testosterone-suppressing therapy.

Premenopause

If you have menstrual periods, you are in premenopause. In premenopause, the ovaries are the main source of estrogen and progesterone. Menstrual periods may stop during treatment and for up to 2 years after treatment, but often returns in those 35 years of age and under.

- Tamoxifen is the endocrine treatment option for those in premenopause. Ovarian suppression or ablation is frequently considered for higher risk ER+ breast cancers.

Menopause

In menopause, the ovaries permanently stop producing hormones and menstrual periods stop. Estrogen and progesterone levels are low, but the adrenal glands, liver, and body fat continue to make small amounts of estrogen. If you don't have periods, a test using a blood sample may be used to confirm your status.

Cancer treatment can cause a temporary menopause. If you stopped having periods due to removal of your uterus (hysterectomy) but you still have your ovaries, then you should have your menopausal status confirmed with a blood test. If both ovaries have been removed (with or without your uterus), you are in menopause.

- Tamoxifen or an aromatase inhibitor is the endocrine treatment for those in menopause. Aromatase inhibitors include anastrozole (Arimidex), exemestane (Aromasin), and letrozole (Femara).

Preventing pregnancy during treatment

If you become pregnant during radiation therapy or endocrine therapy, it can cause birth defects. Use birth control without hormones. Condoms are an option. Speak to your care team about preventing pregnancy while being treated for DCIS.

Clinical trials

A clinical trial is a type of medical research study. After being developed and tested in a laboratory, potential new ways of treating cancer need to be studied in people. If found to be safe and effective in a clinical trial, a drug, device, or treatment approach may be approved by the U.S. Food and Drug Administration (FDA).

Everyone with cancer should carefully consider all of the treatment options available for their cancer type, including standard treatments and clinical trials. Talk to your doctor about whether a clinical trial may make sense for you.

Phases

Most cancer clinical trials focus on treatment. Treatment trials are done in phases.

- **Phase I trials** study the dose, safety, and side effects of an investigational drug or treatment approach. They also look for early signs that the drug or approach is helpful.
- **Phase II trials** study how well the drug or approach works against a specific type of cancer.
- **Phase III trials** test the drug or approach against a standard treatment. If the results are good, it may be approved by the FDA.
- **Phase IV trials** study the long-term safety and benefit of an FDA-approved treatment.

Who can enroll?

Every clinical trial has rules for joining, called eligibility criteria. The rules may be about age, cancer type and stage, treatment history, or general health. These requirements ensure that participants are alike in specific ways and that the trial is as safe as possible for the participants.

Informed consent

Clinical trials are managed by a group of experts called a research team. The research team will review the study with you in detail, including its purpose and the risks and benefits of joining. All of this information is also provided in an informed consent form. Read the form carefully and ask questions before signing it. Take time to discuss with family, friends, or others whom you trust. Keep in mind that you can leave and seek treatment outside of the clinical trial at any time.

Start the conversation

Don't wait for your doctor to bring up clinical trials. Start the conversation and learn about all of your treatment options. If you find a study that you may be eligible for, ask your treatment team if you meet the requirements. If you have already started standard treatment you may not be eligible for certain clinical trials. Try not to be discouraged if you cannot join. New clinical trials are always becoming available.

Frequently asked questions

There are many myths and misconceptions surrounding clinical trials. The possible benefits and risks are not well understood by many with cancer.

Will I get a placebo?

Placebos (inactive versions of real medicines) are almost never used alone in cancer clinical trials. It is common to receive either a placebo with a standard treatment, or a new drug with a standard treatment. You will be informed, verbally and in writing, if a placebo is part of a clinical trial before you enroll.

Do I have to pay to be in a clinical trial?

Rarely. It depends on the study, your health insurance, and the state in which you live. Your treatment team and the research team can help determine if you are responsible for any costs.

Finding a clinical trial

In the United States

NCCN Cancer Centers
NCCN.org/cancercenters

The National Cancer Institute (NCI)
cancer.gov/about-cancer/treatment/clinical-trials/search

Worldwide

The U.S. National Library of Medicine (NLM)
clinicaltrials.gov

Need help finding a clinical trial?

NCI's Cancer Information Service (CIS)
1.800.4.CANCER (1.800.422.6237)
cancer.gov/contact

Supportive care

Supportive care will be specific to your needs. Supportive care is health care given to prevent, reduce, and relieve suffering, and to improve quality of life. Supportive care might include pain relief, palliative care, emotional or spiritual support, financial aid, or family counseling. Tell your care team how you are feeling and about any side effects so they can be managed. Supportive care, best supportive care, and palliative care often mean the same thing.

It is very important to take care of yourself by eating well, drinking plenty of fluids, exercising, and doing things that make you feel energized.

Difficulty eating

Sometimes side effects from surgery, cancer, or other treatments might cause you to feel not hungry or sick to your stomach (nauseated). Healthy eating is important during treatment. It includes eating a balanced diet, eating the right amount of food, and drinking enough fluids. A registered dietitian who is an expert in nutrition and food can help. Speak to your care team if you have trouble eating or maintaining your weight.

Distress

Depression, anxiety, and sleeping issues are common and are a normal part of cancer diagnosis. Talk to your care team and with those whom you feel most comfortable about how you are feeling. There are services, people, and medicine that can help you. Support and counseling services are available.

Fatigue

Fatigue is extreme tiredness and inability to function due to lack of energy. Fatigue may be caused by cancer or it may be a side effect of treatment. Let your care team know how you are feeling and if fatigue is getting in the way of doing the things you enjoy. Eating a balanced diet, exercise, yoga, acupuncture, and massage therapy can help. You might be referred to a nutritionist or dietitian to help with fatigue.

Lymphedema

Lymphedema is a condition in which lymph fluid builds up in tissues and causes swelling. It may be caused when part of the lymph system is damaged or blocked, such as during surgery to remove lymph nodes, or by radiation therapy. Cancers that block lymph vessels can also cause lymphedema. Swelling usually develops slowly over time. It may develop during treatment, or it may start years after treatment. If you have lymphedema, you may be referred to an expert in lymphedema management. The swelling may be reduced by exercise, massage, compression devices, and other means.

Pain

Tell your care team about any pain or discomfort you are having. You might meet with a palliative care specialist or with a pain specialist to manage your pain.

Side effects

All cancer treatments can cause unwanted health issues called side effects. Side effects depend on many factors. These factors include the drug type and dose, length of treatment, and the person. Some side effects may be harmful to your health. Others may just be unpleasant.

Ask for a complete list of side effects of your treatments. Also, tell your treatment team about any new or worsening symptoms. There may be ways to help you feel better. There are also ways to prevent some side effects.

Survivorship

A person is a cancer survivor from the time of diagnosis until the end of life. After treatment, your health will be monitored for side effects of treatment and the return of cancer. This is part of your survivorship care plan. It is important to keep any follow-up doctor visits and imaging test appointments. Seek good routine medical care, including regular doctor visits for preventive care and cancer screening.

A personalized survivorship care plan will contain a summary of possible long-term effects of treatment called late effects and list follow-up tests. Find out how your primary care provider will coordinate with specialists for your follow-up care.

Supportive care resources

More information on supportive care is available at:
NCCN.org/patientguidelines and on the NCCN Patient Guides for Cancer app.

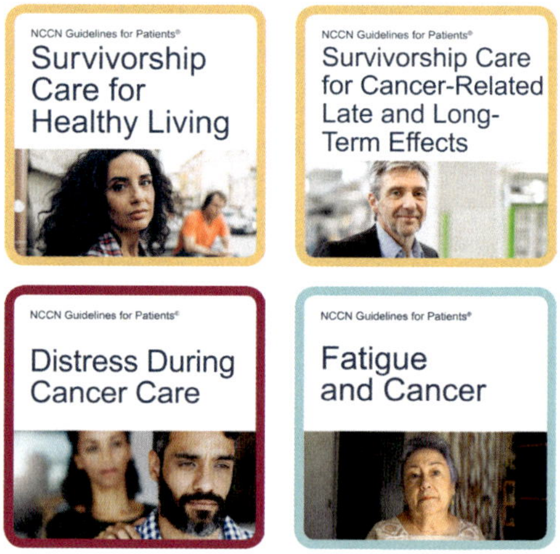

Key points

- Surgery is the main treatment for DCIS. This is only one part of a treatment plan.
- Radiation therapy (RT) uses high-energy radiation from x-rays (photons), electrons, protons, and other sources to kill cancer cells.
- Some breast cancers grow because of estrogen. These cancers are estrogen receptor-positive (ER+) and are often treated with endocrine therapy to reduce the risk of cancer recurrence.
- A clinical trial is a type of research that studies a treatment to see how safe it is and how well it works.
- Supportive care is health care that relieves symptoms caused by treatment and improves quality of life. Supportive care is always given.
- All cancer treatments can cause unwanted health issues called side effects. It is important for you to tell your care team about all your side effects so they can be managed.
- Eating a balanced diet, drinking enough fluids, and exercise can help manage side effects.

Keep a pain diary

A pain diary is a written record that helps you keep track of when you have pain, how bad it is, what causes it, and what makes it better or worse. Use a pain diary to discuss your pain with your care team. You might be referred to a specialist for pain management.

Include in your pain diary:

- ✓ The time and dose of all medicines
- ✓ When pain starts and ends or lessens
- ✓ Where you feel pain
- ✓ A description of your pain. Is it throbbing, sharp, tingling, shooting, or burning? Is it constant, or does it come and go?
- ✓ Does the pain change at different times of day? When?
- ✓ Does the pain get worse before or after meals? Does certain food or drink make it better?
- ✓ Does the pain get better or worse with activity? What kind of activity?
- ✓ Does the pain keep you from falling asleep at night? Does pain wake you up in the night?
- ✓ A rating of your pain from 0 (no pain) to 10 (worst pain you have ever felt)
- ✓ Does pain get in the way of you doing the things you enjoy?

4

Your treatment options

33 Overview

34 Lumpectomy options

34 Mastectomy option

36 Endocrine therapy after lumpectomy

37 Follow-up care

38 Key points

DCIS is treated with surgery. The goal of treatment is to reduce the risk of DCIS progressing to invasive breast cancer. Together, you and your care team will choose a treatment plan that is best for you.

Overview

Ductal carcinoma in situ (DCIS) is treatable. Surgery is a central part of treatment for DCIS. Talk to your care team about what to expect from treatment. Your preferences about treatment are important. Make your wishes known. Treatment options are found in **Guide 2.**

There are 2 types of treatment:

- **Local therapy** focuses on the breast and armpit (axilla) only. It includes surgery and radiation therapy (RT).
- **Systemic therapy** works throughout the body. It includes endocrine therapy. Chemotherapy is not used to treat DCIS.

The goal of treatment is to prevent DCIS from growing outside the duct into surrounding tissue. When cancer spreads into the surrounding tissue, it is called invasive breast cancer. Invasive breast cancer is breast cancer that has spread from the milk ducts or milk glands (lobules) into the breast tissue or to nearby lymph nodes.

Guide 2 Treatment options
Option 1
• Lumpectomy with whole breast radiation therapy (WBRT) • Lumpectomy with WBRT and radiation boost
Option 2
• Lumpectomy with accelerated partial breast irradiation (APBI) or partial breast irradiation (PBI)
Option 3
• Lumpectomy only (not an option for most people)
Option 4
• Total mastectomy with sentinel lymph node biopsy (SLNB) • Flat closure or reconstruction after mastectomy

Lumpectomy options

A lumpectomy is also known as breast-conserving surgery (BCS). It may or may not be followed by radiation therapy. Lymph node surgery is not done with a lumpectomy. You may have more than one surgery to ensure all the cancer was removed.

A lumpectomy followed by radiation therapy is an option for many but not all with DCIS. This is not an option if you are pregnant, have some health issues, or the cancer is throughout the breast. The surgical margin must be cancer-free, called a negative surgical margin (R0). Lumpectomy options are described next.

Lumpectomy with whole breast radiation therapy

Most of your breast will be treated with radiation in whole breast radiation therapy (WBRT). Whole breast radiation will help to prevent the return of cancer. For every cancer that returns there is an equal chance of developing DCIS again or an invasive type of cancer. Many factors are used to determine risk of recurrence. Ask your care team if your risk of cancer coming back is low or high. If it's high, you may receive extra radiation called a boost.

Lumpectomy with partial breast radiation therapy

When radiation therapy (RT) is given only to the lumpectomy site, it is called partial breast irradiation (PBI). This is an option in some cases. You must have a low risk of the cancer returning. Surgical margins must be cancer-free. The size, grade, and other features of the tumor will be considered. Accelerated partial breast irradiation (APBI) therapy is radiation given over a shorter length of time.

Lumpectomy only

Treatment with a lumpectomy only (no radiation) is an option for a small group of people. You must have a low risk of the cancer coming back. Surgical margins must be cancer-free. The size, grade, and other features of the tumor will be considered.

Mastectomy option

A total mastectomy or a simple mastectomy is a surgery that removes the whole breast. Chest muscle is not removed. A skin-sparing mastectomy removes the breast but not all of the skin. A nipple-sparing mastectomy preserves the nipple-areola complex (NAC) and the skin. Not everyone is a candidate for nipple-sparing mastectomy. You might choose to have a flat closure or breast reconstruction after a mastectomy.

There are many reasons why a total mastectomy might be the best choice for you.

- Cancer may be found at the surgical margin.
- The tumor might be large, too big, or widespread.
- You may be at risk of developing a second cancer.
- You might have a health issue.
- You may want a mastectomy.
- You may not be able to receive radiation to the breast area.

Total mastectomy with sentinel lymph node biopsy

A sentinel lymph node biopsy (SLNB) is done at the time of mastectomy. Sentinel lymph nodes are the first lymph nodes cancer cells are likely to have spread to from the primary tumor. An SLNB finds and removes a few of these nodes. The nodes are then tested for cancer. Once the breast is removed, an SLNB can't be done. Instead, many lymph nodes would have to be removed to test for cancer. This is because a mastectomy permanently changes lymph flow and drainage. Therefore, an SLNB will be done at the time of a mastectomy just in case there is a small area of invasive cancer in the breast.

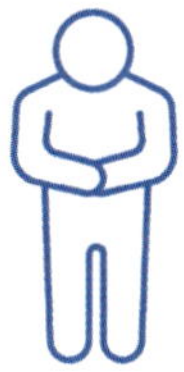

You know your body better than anyone

Help your care team understand:

- ✓ How you feel
- ✓ What you need
- ✓ What is working and what is not

Keep a list of names and contact information for each member of your team. This will make it easier for you and anyone involved in your care to know whom to contact with questions or concerns.

Get to know your care team and help them get to know you.

Endocrine therapy after lumpectomy

Endocrine therapy is often given after a lumpectomy for cancers that are estrogen receptor-positive (ER+). This is given to reduce the risk of cancer returning. For treatment after breast-conserving surgery, **see Guide 3.**

Endocrine therapy

Endocrine therapy includes treatments that stop cancer growth caused by hormones. It is sometimes called hormone therapy. It is not the same as hormone replacement therapy (HRT).

Endocrine therapy may be given to help reduce the risk of developing a second breast cancer in those who were treated with:

- Breast-conserving surgery (lumpectomy) with radiation therapy (RT)
- Lumpectomy alone
- Mastectomy on one side only

There is more than one type of endocrine therapy. The type prescribed by your care team is partly based on if you have menstrual periods.

- Those who have menstrual periods are in premenopause. Tamoxifen is an option.
- Those whose menstrual periods have stopped for more than 12 months are in menopause. Tamoxifen or an aromatase inhibitor (AI) is an option.

While taking endocrine therapy, it is important to have follow-up visits with your care team and seek regular preventive care with a dentist. Let your dentist know if you are taking any of these medicines. Let your care team know about any planned dental procedures.

Medicine might be given to prevent bone loss and fractures while on endocrine therapy. A calcium and vitamin D supplement might be recommended, but talk to your care team first.

Guide 3
Treatment after breast-conserving surgery (lumpectomy)

Consider endocrine therapy for 5 years for those with estrogen receptor-positive (ER+) DCIS if treated with:

- Breast-conserving surgery (lumpectomy) and radiation therapy (RT)
- Lumpectomy alone
- Mastectomy on one side only

Endocrine therapy options:

- For those in premenopause, tamoxifen
- For those in menopause, tamoxifen or aromatase inhibitor (AI)

Follow-up care

After treatment, you will receive follow-up care. It is important to keep any follow-up visits and imaging test appointments. Contact your doctor if you have any new or worsening symptoms.

Medical history and physical exam

An update of your medical history and a physical exam are part of follow-up care. Both should be done every 6 to 12 months for 5 years, then once a year after 5 years of normal results.

Mammogram

A mammogram should be done every 12 months after breast-conserving treatment. If you had both breasts removed to reduce your cancer risk, then mammograms aren't needed.

Lowering your risk

There are things you can do to lower your chance of developing breast cancer in the future. Changes in your lifestyle include eating a mostly plant-based diet, exercising, limiting alcohol, and quitting smoking. Your care team can offer information and support on how to lower your risk.

Take care of yourself. This is a stressful time. Seek out support groups at your local hospital, through social media, or from those listed in the back of this book. Look to friends, relatives, neighbors, and coworkers for social support.

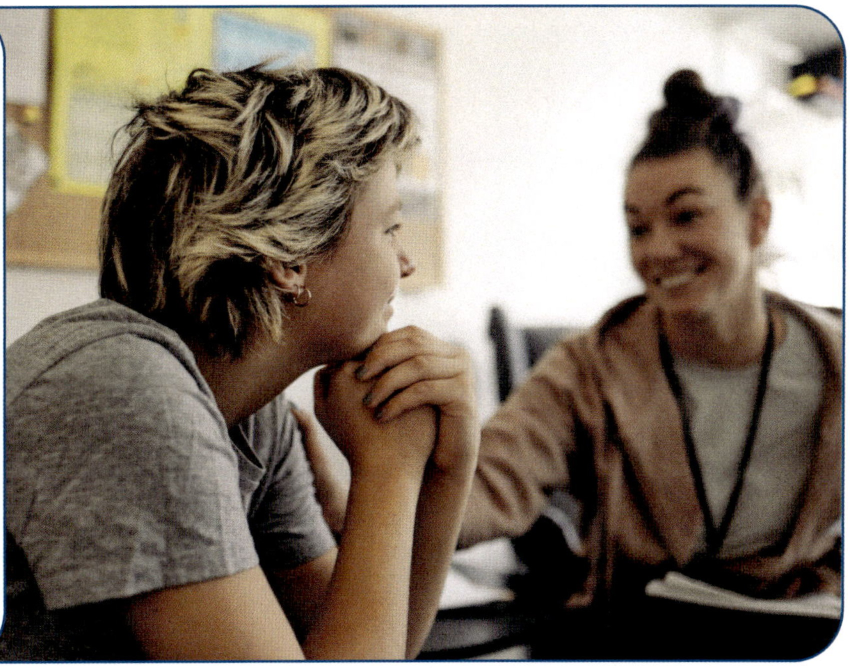

Key points

- Ductal carcinoma in situ (DCIS) is treatable. The goal of treatment is to reduce the risk of DCIS progressing to invasive breast cancer.
- Treatment for DCIS is usually a combination of surgery and radiation therapy followed by endocrine therapy.
- Surgery options include a lumpectomy or mastectomy. A lumpectomy is also called breast-conserving surgery (BCS) or partial mastectomy.
- Local therapy focuses on the breast and armpit (axilla) only. It includes surgery and radiation therapy.
- Systemic therapy works throughout the body. It includes endocrine therapy. Chemotherapy is not used to treat DCIS.
- Lifestyle changes, endocrine therapy, and surgery help to reduce the risk of future breast cancer.
- Follow-up care includes physical exams and mammograms.

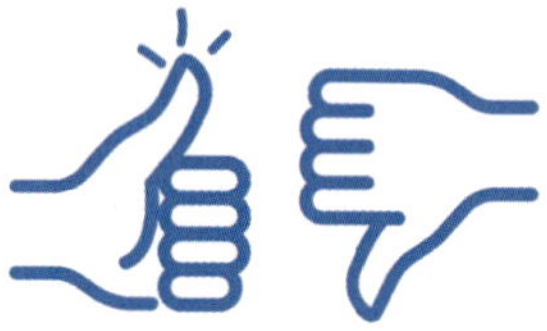

Let us know what you think!

Please take a moment to complete an online survey about the NCCN Guidelines for Patients.

NCCN.org/patients/response

5

The breast after surgery

40 Volume displacement

40 Flat closure

41 Breast reconstruction

43 What to consider

43 Key points

The look of your breast after surgery will depend on the type of surgery, the amount of tissue removed, and other factors such as your body type, age, and size and shape of the area before surgery. You might consider speaking with a plastic surgeon before surgery. This chapter offers more information on volume displacement, flat closure, and breast reconstruction.

The recovery time for each procedure differs. This can affect your ability to return to work or participate in activities. You might consider speaking with a plastic surgeon before surgery to discuss your options and what to expect.

Volume displacement

With a lumpectomy, most people have a scar with some volume loss. However, if you need a large lumpectomy and your surgeon thinks your breast will look more abnormal afterwards, your breast may be able to be re-shaped at the time of surgery. This procedure is called volume displacement or oncoplasty. Only a limited number of cancer centers perform this procedure. It is often done by the cancer surgeon or plastic surgeon right after the lumpectomy. The surgeon will shift the remaining breast tissue to fill the space left by the removed tumor.

If volume displacement is planned, a larger piece of your breast will need to be removed. Despite a larger piece being removed, the natural look of your breast will be kept. However, with large amounts of tissue removed, your breast may be smaller than before.

You may not like the results of the volume displacement. In this case, breast revision surgery may help. This surgery is done by a plastic surgeon. A second volume displacement may be an option, too. Another option is to get breast implants or mastectomy with reconstruction.

Flat closure

In a total mastectomy with a flat closure, the entire breast, including nipple, extra skin, fat, and other tissue in the breast area, is removed. The remaining skin is tightened and sewn together. No breast mound is created, and no implant is added. The scar will be slightly raised and differ in color than the surrounding skin. A flat closure is not completely flat or smooth. The result varies from person to person. Ask to look at pictures from flat closures so you know what to expect.

You might decide to have a flat closure procedure later or after having breast implants removed. Talk to your care team to learn more.

Breast reconstruction

Breast reconstruction is surgery to rebuild the shape and look of the breast after a mastectomy. In many cases, breast reconstruction involves a staged approach. It might require more than one procedure.

You may have a choice as to when breast reconstruction is done. Immediate reconstruction is finished within hours after removing the breast. Delayed reconstruction can occur months or years after the cancer surgery. Reconstruction can also be done in a staged fashion, with part of the reconstruction done at the time of the original cancer surgery and finished with another surgery later. A plastic surgeon performs breast reconstruction.

Breasts can be reconstructed with implants and flaps. All methods are generally safe, but as with any surgery, there are risks. Ask your treatment team for a complete list of side effects.

Implants

Breast implants are small bags filled with salt water, silicone gel, or both. They are placed under the breast skin or muscle to look like a new breast following a mastectomy. A balloon-like device, called an expander, may be used first to stretch out tissue. It will be placed under your skin or muscle and enlarged every few weeks for 2 to 3 months. When your skin is stretched to the proper size, you will have surgery to place the final implant.

Implants have a small risk of leaking or causing other issues. You may feel pain from the implant or expander. Scar tissue or tissue death can occur.

Your preferences about treatment are always important. Talk to your care team and make your wishes known.

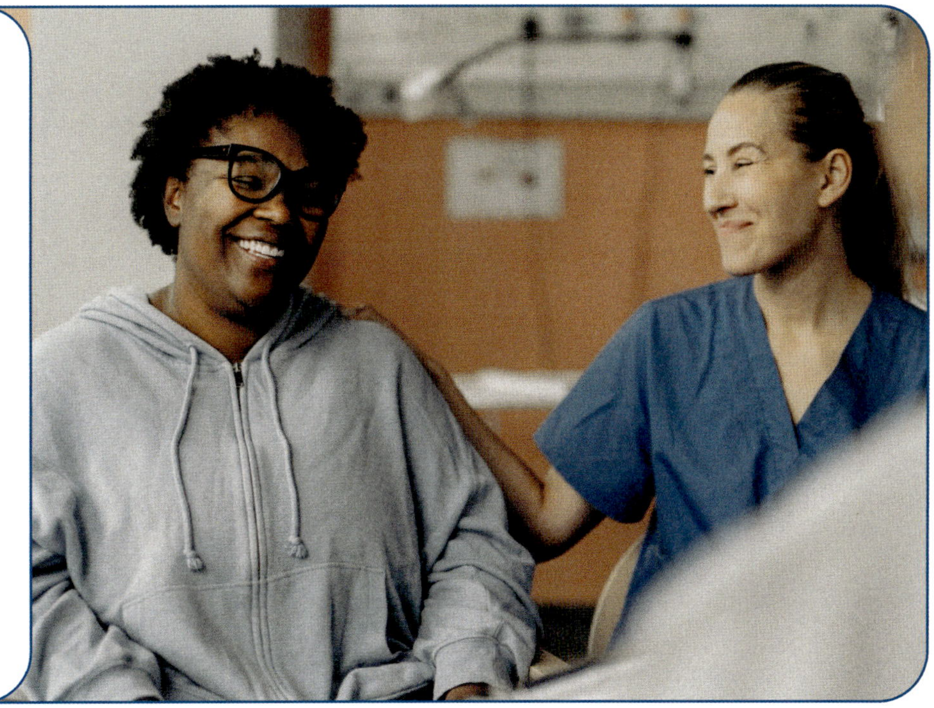

Flaps

Sometimes breast fullness can be recreated after a skin-sparing mastectomy. In a skin-sparing mastectomy, breast tissue is removed from underneath the skin. The nipple remains intact, if possible. The remaining skin flaps are used to create a breast mound. This technique does not use implants or skin transferred from other parts of the body and may be completed in a single surgery. This technique, called a Goldilocks mastectomy, is best suited for those with larger breasts who are willing to have much smaller breasts as a result.

Breasts can be remade using tissue from other parts of your body, known as flaps. These flaps are taken from the abdomen, buttocks, thigh, or from under the shoulder blade. Some flaps are completely removed and then sewn in place. Other flaps stay attached to your body but are slid over and sewn into place.

There are several risks associated with flaps, including death of fat in the flap, which can cause lumps. A hernia may result from muscle weakness. Problems are more likely to occur among those who have diabetes or who smoke.

Implants and flaps

Some breasts are reconstructed with both implants and flaps. This method may give the reconstructed breast more volume to match the other breast. For any reconstruction, you may need surgery on your remaining breast to match the two breasts in size and shape.

Nipple replacement

Like your breast, a nipple can be remade. To rebuild a nipple, a plastic surgeon can use surrounding tissues. Also, nipples can be remade with tissue from the thigh or other nipple. Tissue can be darkened with a tattoo to look more like a nipple. It is important to note that while you can remake something to look like a nipple, it will not have the sensation of your real nipple. Also, a tattoo can be done to look like a nipple without having to take tissue from another part of the body.

What to consider

Some things to consider when deciding to have flat closure or reconstruction after mastectomy:

- **Your desire –** You may have a strong feeling towards flat closure or one form of reconstruction after being given the options. Breast reconstruction should be a shared decision between you and your care team. Make your wishes known.
- **Health issues –** You may have health issues such as diabetes or a blood disorder that might affect or delay healing, or make longer procedures unsafe.
- **Tobacco use –** Smoking delays wound healing and can cause mastectomy flap death (necrosis), nipple-areola complex (NAC) necrosis in a nipple-sparing mastectomy, infection, and failure of implant-based reconstruction. In free flap reconstruction, smoking increases the risk of complications. You are encouraged to stop smoking prior to reconstruction.
- **Breast size and shape –** There are limits to the available sizes of breast implants. Very large breasts or breasts that lack tone or droop (called ptosis) might be difficult to match. Breast reduction surgery might be an option.
- **Body mass index (BMI) –** Those with an elevated BMI have an increased risk of infections and complications with breast reconstruction.

Key points

- Volume displacement is a shifting of the breast tissue to fill the space left by a lumpectomy.
- Flat closure is done after a mastectomy in which the skin is tightened and sewn together without the addition of a breast implant.
- Breast reconstruction is surgery to rebuild the shape and look of the breast.
- Breasts that are fully removed in a mastectomy can be remade with breast implants, flaps, or both.
- Removed nipples can be remade with body tissue and/or tattooing.

6
Making treatment decisions

45 It's your choice

45 Questions to ask

53 Resources

It's important to be comfortable with the cancer treatment you choose. This choice starts with having an open and honest conversation with your care team.

It's your choice

In shared decision-making, you and your team share information, discuss the options, and agree on a treatment plan. It starts with an open and honest conversation between you and your care team.

Treatment decisions are very personal. What is important to you may not be important to someone else.

Some things that may play a role in your decision-making:

- What you want and how that might differ from what others want
- Your religious and spiritual beliefs
- Your feelings about certain treatments
- Your feelings about pain or side effects
- Cost of treatment, travel to treatment centers, and time away from school, work, and family
- Quality of life and length of life
- How active you are and the activities that are important to you

Think about what you want from treatment. Discuss openly the risks and benefits of specific treatments and procedures. Weigh options and share concerns with your care team. If you take the time to build a relationship with your care team, it will help you feel supported when considering options and making treatment decisions.

Second opinion

It is normal to want to start treatment as soon as possible. While cancer can't be ignored, there is time to have another doctor review your test results and suggest a treatment plan. This is called getting a second opinion, and it's a normal part of cancer care. Even doctors get second opinions!

Things you can do to prepare:

- Check with your insurance company about its rules on second opinions. There may be out-of-pocket costs to see doctors who are not part of your insurance plan.
- Make plans to have copies of all your records sent to the doctor you will see for your second opinion.

Support groups

Many people diagnosed with cancer find support groups to be helpful. Support groups often include people at different stages of treatment. Some people may be newly diagnosed, while others may be finished with treatment. If your hospital or community doesn't have support groups for people with cancer, check out the websites listed in this book.

Questions to ask

Possible questions to ask your care team are listed on the following pages. Feel free to use these questions or come up with your own. Be clear about your goals for treatment and find out what to expect from treatment.

Questions about testing and diagnosis

1. What tests will I have? How often will they be repeated?
2. Will my insurance pay for this test?
3. What will you do to make me comfortable during testing?
4. What if I am pregnant or want to become pregnant soon?
5. When will I have a biopsy?
6. What are the risks with a biopsy?
7. How will my biopsy be performed?
8. What else might be done during the biopsy?
9. How soon will I know the results and who will explain them to me?
10. How can I get a copy of the pathology report and other test results?

Questions about your care team's experience

1. What is your experience treating DCIS? What else do you treat?
2. What is the experience of those on your team?
3. How many people like me have you treated?
4. Will you be consulting with experts to discuss my care? Whom will you consult?
5. How many procedures like the one you're suggesting have you done?
6. Is this treatment a major part of your practice?
7. How often is a complication expected? What are the complications?
8. How many breast cancer surgeries have you done?
9. Who will manage my day-to-day care?

Questions about options

1. What will happen if I do nothing?
2. Which option is proven to work best for my cancer, age, overall health, and other risk factors?
3. What are the possible complications and side effects? Are any life-threatening?
4. What can be done to prevent or relieve the side effects of treatment?
5. Am I a candidate for a clinical trial?
6. Can I join a clinical trial at any time?
7. What decisions must be made today?
8. Is there a social worker or someone who can help me decide about treatment?
9. Is there a hospital or treatment center you can recommend for breast cancer treatment?
10. Can I go to one hospital for surgery and a different center for radiation therapy?

Questions about treatment

1. Which treatment(s) do you recommend and why?
2. Does the order of treatment matter?
3. When will I start treatment?
4. How long will treatment take?
5. What should I expect from treatment?
6. What will you do to make me comfortable during treatment?
7. How much will my insurance pay for treatment?
8. Are there programs to help me pay for treatment?
9. What are the chances my cancer will return after treatment?
10. I would like a second opinion. Is there someone you can recommend?

Questions about surgery

1. How much of my breast will be removed?
2. What will my breast look like after surgery?
3. What lymph nodes might be removed during surgery?
4. What are the chances you can remove the whole tumor with a negative margin?
5. How can I prepare for surgery?
6. How long will recovery take and what should I expect?
7. When will I be able to return to work or normal activities after surgery?
8. How much pain will I be in and what will be done to manage my pain?
9. What complications can occur from this surgery?
10. What options are available if I do not like the look of my breast after surgery?

Questions about radiation therapy

1. What type of radiation therapy (RT) will I have?
2. What will you target?
3. What is the goal of this RT?
4. How many treatment sessions will I require?
5. Can you do a shorter course of RT?
6. Do you offer this type of RT here? If not, should I be referred to someone who does?
7. What side effects can I expect from RT?
8. Will I be given medicine to help me relax during RT?
9. What should I wear?

Questions about resources and support

1. Who can I talk to about help with housing, food, and other basic needs?
2. What help is available for transportation, childcare, and home care?
3. How much will I have to pay for treatment?
4. What help is available to pay for medicines and other treatment?
5. What other services are available to me and my caregivers?
6. How can I connect with others and build a support system?
7. How can I find in-person or online support?
8. Who can help me with my concerns about missing work or school?
9. Who can I talk to if I don't feel safe at home, at work, or in my neighborhood?
10. How can I get help to stop smoking or vaping?

Resources

Breast Cancer Alliance (BCA)
breastcanceralliance.org

Breastcancer.org
breastcancer.org

Cancer Hope Network
cancerhopenetwork.org

DiepC Foundation
diepcfoundation.org

FORCE: Facing Our Risk of Cancer Empowered
facingourrisk.org

GPAC Global Patient Advocacy Coalition
GPACunited.org

Inflammatory Breast Cancer Research Foundation
ibcresearch.org

Lobular Breast Cancer Alliance
lobularbreastcancer.org

MedlinePlus
medlineplus.gov/breastcancer.html

National Cancer Institute (NCI)
cancer.gov/types/breast

National Coalition for Cancer Survivorship
canceradvocacy.org

Sharsheret
sharsheret.org

Triage Cancer
triagecancer.org

Unite for HER
uniteforher.org

Words to know

accelerated partial breast irradiation (APBI)
Treatment with radiation to the part of the breast with cancer. It is often given over a shorter period of time compared to whole breast radiation therapy.

anti-estrogen
A drug that stops estrogen from attaching to cells.

areola
A darker, round area of skin on the breast around the nipple.

aromatase inhibitor (AI)
A drug that lowers the level of estrogen in the body.

bilateral diagnostic mammogram
Pictures of the insides of both breasts that are made from a set of x-rays.

biopsy
A procedure that removes fluid or tissue samples to be tested for a disease.

boost
An extra dose of radiation to a specific area of the body.

breast-conserving surgery (BCS)
A cancer treatment that includes removing a breast lump.

breast implant
A small bag filled with salt water, gel, or both that is used to remake breasts.

breast reconstruction
An operation that creates new breasts.

cancer stage
A rating of the outlook of a cancer based on its growth and spread.

carcinoma
A cancer of cells that line the inner or outer surfaces of the body.

chest wall
The layer of muscle, bone, and fat that protects the vital organs.

clinical breast exam (CBE)
Touching of a breast by a health expert to feel for diseases.

clinical stage (c)
The rating of the extent of cancer before treatment is started.

clinical trial
A type of research that assesses health tests or treatments.

connective tissue
Supporting and binding tissue that surrounds other tissues and organs.

contrast
A substance put into your body to make clearer pictures during imaging tests.

core needle biopsy (CNB)
A procedure that removes tissue samples with a hollow needle. Also called core biopsy.

diagnostic bilateral mammogram
Pictures of the insides of both breasts that are made from a set of x-rays.

duct
A tube-shaped structure through which milk travels to the nipple.

ductal carcinoma in situ (DCIS)
A breast cancer that has not grown outside the breast ducts.

endocrine therapy
A cancer treatment that stops the making or action of estrogen. Also called hormone therapy.

estrogen
A hormone that plays a role in breast development.

estrogen receptor (ER)
A protein inside cells that binds to estrogen.

estrogen receptor-negative (ER-)
A type of breast cancer that doesn't use estrogen to grow.

estrogen receptor-positive (ER+)
A type of breast cancer that uses estrogen to grow.

fine-needle aspiration (FNA)
A procedure that removes tissue samples with a very thin needle.

flat closure
Procedure done after a mastectomy in which the skin is tightened and sewn together without the addition of a breast implant.

gene
Coded instructions in cells for making new cells and controlling how cells behave.

genetic counseling
Expert guidance on the chance for a disease that is passed down in families.

hereditary breast cancer
Breast cancer likely caused by abnormal genes passed down from biological parent to child.

histology
The structure of cells, tissue, and organs as viewed under a microscope.

hormone
A chemical in the body that triggers a response from cells or organs.

immunohistochemistry (IHC)
A lab test of cancer cells to find specific cell traits involved in abnormal cell growth.

invasive breast cancer
The growth of breast cancer into the breast's supporting tissue (stroma).

lobule
A gland in the breast that makes breast milk.

lumpectomy
An operation that removes a small breast cancer tumor. Also called breast-conserving surgery.

lymph
A clear fluid containing white blood cells.

lymph node
A small, bean-shaped disease-fighting structure.

lymphadenopathy
Lymph nodes that are abnormal in size or consistency.

lymphatic system
Germ-fighting network of tissues and organs that includes the bone marrow, spleen, thymus, lymph nodes, and lymphatic vessels. Part of the immune system.

lymphedema
Swelling in the body caused by a buildup of fluid called lymph.

magnetic resonance imaging (MRI)
A test that uses radio waves and powerful magnets to make pictures of the insides of the body.

mammogram
A picture of the insides of the breast that is made using x-rays.

mastectomy
An operation that removes the whole breast.

medical history
A report of all your health events and medications.

menopause
The point in time 12 months after a last menstrual period.

mutation
An abnormal change.

nipple-areola complex (NAC)
The ring of darker breast skin is called the areola. The raised tip within the areola is called the nipple.

noninvasive breast cancer
Breast cancer that has not grown into tissue from which it can spread.

palpable adenopathy
Lymph nodes that feel abnormal in size or consistency.

partial breast irradiation (PBI)
Treatment with radiation that is received at the site of the removed breast tumor.

pathologic stage (p)
A rating of the extent of cancer given after examining tissue removed during surgery.

pathologist
A doctor who's an expert in testing cells and tissue to find disease.

postmenopause
The state of having no more menstrual periods.

premenopause
The state of having menstrual periods.

primary tumor
The first mass of cancer cells.

prognosis
The likely course and outcome of a disease based on tests.

radiation therapy (RT)
A treatment that uses high-energy rays. Also called radiotherapy.

recurrence
The return of cancer after a cancer-free period.

sentinel lymph node (SLN)
The first lymph node to which cancer cells spread after leaving a tumor.

sentinel lymph node biopsy (SLNB)
An operation to remove the disease-fighting structures (lymph nodes) to which cancer first spreads. Also called sentinel lymph node dissection.

side effect
An unhealthy or unpleasant physical or emotional response to treatment.

skin-sparing mastectomy
An operation that removes all breast tissue but saves as much breast skin as possible.

supportive care
Health care that includes symptom relief but not cancer treatment. Also called palliative care or best supportive care.

surgical margin
The normal-looking tissue around a tumor removed during an operation.

systemic therapy
Drug treatment that works throughout the body.

total mastectomy
An operation that removes the entire breast with a flat closure. Also called simple mastectomy.

ultrasound (US)
A test that uses sound waves to take pictures of the inside of the body.

vacuum-assisted core biopsy (VACB)
A procedure in which a small sample of tissue is removed from the breast with the aid of a vacuum device.

volume displacement
A method to shift breast tissue during an operation to fill a space left from a lumpectomy.

whole breast radiation therapy (WBRT)
Treatment with radiation of the entire breast.

share with us.

Take our survey and help make the NCCN Guidelines for Patients better for everyone!

NCCN.org/patients/comments

NCCN Contributors

This patient guide is based on the NCCN Clinical Practice Guidelines in Oncology (NCCN Guidelines®) for Breast Cancer, Version 1.2024. It was adapted, reviewed, and published with help from the following people:

Dorothy A. Shead, MS
Senior Director
Patient Information Operations

Tanya Fischer, MEd, MSLIS
Senior Medical Writer

Susan Kidney
Senior Graphic Design Specialist

The NCCN Clinical Practice Guidelines in Oncology (NCCN Guidelines®) for Breast Cancer, Version 1.2024 were developed by the following NCCN Panel Members:

William J. Gradishar, MD/Chair
Robert H. Lurie Comprehensive Cancer Center of Northwestern University

Meena S. Moran, MD/Vice-Chair
Yale Cancer Center/Smilow Cancer Hospital

Jame Abraham, MD
Case Comprehensive Cancer Center/ University Hospitals Seidman Cancer Center and Cleveland Clinic Taussig Cancer Institute

Vandana Abramson, MD
Vanderbilt-Ingram Cancer Center

*Rebecca Aft, MD, PhD
Siteman Cancer Center at Barnes-Jewish Hospital and Washington University School of Medicine

Doreen Agnese, MD
The Ohio State University Comprehensive Cancer Center - James Cancer Hospital and Solove Research Institute

Kimberly H. Allison, MD
Stanford Cancer Institute

*Bethany Anderson, MD
University of Wisconsin Carbone Cancer Center

Janet Bailey, MD
University of Michigan Rogel Cancer Center

Harold J. Burstein, MD, PhD
Dana-Farber/Brigham and Women's Cancer Center

Nan Chen, MD
The UChicago Medicine Comprehensive Cancer Center

Helen Chew, MD
UC Davis Comprehensive Cancer Center

Chau Dang, MD
Memorial Sloan Kettering Cancer Center

Anthony D. Elias, MD
University of Colorado Cancer Center

Sharon H. Giordano, MD, MPH
The University of Texas MD Anderson Cancer Center

Matthew P. Goetz, MD
Mayo Clinic Comprehensive Cancer Center

Rachel C. Jankowitz, MD
Abramson Cancer Center at the University of Pennsylvania

Sara H. Javid, MD
Fred Hutchinson Cancer Center

Jairam Krishnamurthy, MD
Fred & Pamela Buffett Cancer Center

A. Marilyn Leitch, MD
UT Southwestern Simmons Comprehensive Cancer Center

Janice Lyons, MD
Case Comprehensive Cancer Center/ University Hospitals Seidman Cancer Center and Cleveland Clinic Taussig Cancer Institute

Susie McCloskey, MD, MSHS
UCLA Jonsson Comprehensive Cancer Center

Melissa McShane, MD
Fox Chase Cancer Center

Joanne Mortimer, MD
City of Hope National Medical Center

Sameer A. Patel, MD
Fox Chase Cancer Center

Laura H. Rosenberger, MD, MS
Duke Cancer Institute

Hope S. Rugo, MD
UCSF Helen Diller Family Comprehensive Cancer Center

Cesar Santa-Maria, MD, MSCI
The Sidney Kimmel Comprehensive Cancer Center at Johns Hopkins

Bryan P. Schneider, MD
Indiana University Melvin and Bren Simon Comprehensive Cancer Center

*Mary Lou Smith, JD, MBA
Research Advocacy Network

Hatem Soliman, MD
Moffitt Cancer Center

Erica M. Stringer-Reasor, MD
O'Neal Comprehensive Cancer Center at UAB

Melinda L. Telli, MD
Stanford Cancer Institute

Mei Wei, MD
Huntsman Cancer Institute at the University of Utah

Kari B. Wisinski, MD
University of Wisconsin Carbone Cancer Center

Kay T. Yeung, MD, PhD
UC San Diego Moores Cancer Center

*Jessica S. Young, MD
Roswell Park Comprehensive Cancer Center

NCCN

Rashmi Kumar, PhD
Senior Director, Clinical Content

Ryan Schonfeld, BA
Guidelines Coordinator

* Reviewed this patient guide. For disclosures, visit NCCN.org/disclosures.

NCCN Cancer Centers

Abramson Cancer Center
at the University of Pennsylvania
Philadelphia, Pennsylvania
800.789.7366 • pennmedicine.org/cancer

Case Comprehensive Cancer Center/
University Hospitals Seidman Cancer Center and
Cleveland Clinic Taussig Cancer Institute
Cleveland, Ohio
UH Seidman Cancer Center
800.641.2422 • uhhospitals.org/services/cancer-services
CC Taussig Cancer Institute
866.223.8100 • my.clevelandclinic.org/departments/cancer
Case CCC
216.844.8797 • case.edu/cancer

City of Hope National Medical Center
Duarte, California
800.826.4673 • cityofhope.org

Dana-Farber/Brigham and Women's Cancer Center |
Mass General Cancer Center
Boston, Massachusetts
617.732.5500 • youhaveus.org
617.726.5130 • massgeneral.org/cancer-center

Duke Cancer Institute
Durham, North Carolina
888.275.3853 • dukecancerinstitute.org

Fox Chase Cancer Center
Philadelphia, Pennsylvania
888.369.2427 • foxchase.org

Fred & Pamela Buffett Cancer Center
Omaha, Nebraska
402.559.5600 • unmc.edu/cancercenter

Fred Hutchinson Cancer Center
Seattle, Washington
206.667.5000 • fredhutch.org

Huntsman Cancer Institute at the University of Utah
Salt Lake City, Utah
800.824.2073 • healthcare.utah.edu/huntsmancancerinstitute

Indiana University Melvin and Bren Simon
Comprehensive Cancer Center
Indianapolis, Indiana
888.600.4822 • www.cancer.iu.edu

Mayo Clinic Comprehensive Cancer Center
Phoenix/Scottsdale, Arizona
Jacksonville, Florida
Rochester, Minnesota
480.301.8000 • Arizona
904.953.0853 • Florida
507.538.3270 • Minnesota
mayoclinic.org/cancercenter

Memorial Sloan Kettering Cancer Center
New York, New York
800.525.2225 • mskcc.org

Moffitt Cancer Center
Tampa, Florida
888.663.3488 • moffitt.org

O'Neal Comprehensive Cancer Center at UAB
Birmingham, Alabama
800.822.0933 • uab.edu/onealcancercenter

Robert H. Lurie Comprehensive Cancer Center
of Northwestern University
Chicago, Illinois
866.587.4322 • cancer.northwestern.edu

Roswell Park Comprehensive Cancer Center
Buffalo, New York
877.275.7724 • roswellpark.org

Siteman Cancer Center at Barnes-Jewish Hospital
and Washington University School of Medicine
St. Louis, Missouri
800.600.3606 • siteman.wustl.edu

St. Jude Children's Research Hospital/
The University of Tennessee Health Science Center
Memphis, Tennessee
866.278.5833 • stjude.org
901.448.5500 • uthsc.edu

Stanford Cancer Institute
Stanford, California
877.668.7535 • cancer.stanford.edu

The Ohio State University Comprehensive Cancer Center -
James Cancer Hospital and Solove Research Institute
Columbus, Ohio
800.293.5066 • cancer.osu.edu

The Sidney Kimmel Comprehensive
Cancer Center at Johns Hopkins
Baltimore, Maryland
410.955.8964
www.hopkinskimmelcancercenter.org

The UChicago Medicine Comprehensive Cancer Center
Chicago, Illinois
773.702.1000 • uchicagomedicine.org/cancer

The University of Texas MD Anderson Cancer Center
Houston, Texas
844.269.5922 • mdanderson.org

UC Davis Comprehensive Cancer Center
Sacramento, California
916.734.5959 • 800.770.9261
health.ucdavis.edu/cancer

UC San Diego Moores Cancer Center
La Jolla, California
858.822.6100 • *cancer.ucsd.edu*

UCLA Jonsson Comprehensive Cancer Center
Los Angeles, California
310.825.5268 • *uclahealth.org/cancer*

UCSF Helen Diller Family Comprehensive Cancer Center
San Francisco, California
800.689.8273 • *cancer.ucsf.edu*

University of Colorado Cancer Center
Aurora, Colorado
720.848.0300 • *coloradocancercenter.org*

University of Michigan Rogel Cancer Center
Ann Arbor, Michigan
800.865.1125 • *rogelcancercenter.org*

University of Wisconsin Carbone Cancer Center
Madison, Wisconsin
608.265.1700 • *uwhealth.org/cancer*

UT Southwestern Simmons Comprehensive Cancer Center
Dallas, Texas
214.648.3111 • *utsouthwestern.edu/simmons*

Vanderbilt-Ingram Cancer Center
Nashville, Tennessee
877.936.8422 • *vicc.org*

Yale Cancer Center/Smilow Cancer Hospital
New Haven, Connecticut
855.4.SMILOW • *yalecancercenter.org*

We want your feedback!

Our goal is to provide helpful and easy-to-understand information on cancer.

Take our survey to let us know what we got right and what we could do better.

NCCN.org/patients/feedback

Index

accelerated partial breast irradiation (APBI) 24, 34

biopsy 12–13

birth control 26

BRCA 15

breast-conserving surgery (BCS) 34

breast reconstruction 41–42

breastfeeding 23

cancer stages 16–17

chestfeeding 23

clinical breast exam (CBE) 10

clinical trials 27–28

clips or markers 13

contrast 11

diagnostic mammogram 7, 11

ductal carcinoma in situ (DCIS) 6

endocrine therapy 25–26, 36

estrogen 14, 25

estrogen receptor (ER) 14

family history 10, 15

flat closure 40

genetic testing 15

hereditary breast cancer 15

hormone therapy (see endocrine therapy)

lumpectomy 34

magnetic resonance imaging (MRI) 11

mammogram 7, 11

mastectomy 34–35

menopause 26

menstruation 26

nipple replacement 42

partial breast irradiation (PBI) 24, 34

pregnancy 26

premenopause 26

radiation therapy (RT) 24

sentinel lymph node biopsy (SLNB) 24, 35

supportive care 29–30

surgery 22–24

survivorship 30, 37

testosterone 26

those assigned male at birth 6, 26

TNM scores 16

ultrasound 11

volume displacement 40

whole breast radiation therapy (WBRT) 24, 34

Made in the USA
Monee, IL
20 November 2024

70672550R00038